Asthma

The Concise Guide on How to Manage your Asthma Symptoms in a time of Viral Outbreak & Pandemic

Melinda Perry

Copyright © 2020 Melinda Perry

All rights reserved. No part of this publication may be reproduced, distributed, or transmitted in any form or by any means, including photocopying, recording, or other electronic or mechanical methods, without the prior written permission of the publisher, except in the case of brief quotations embodied in critical reviews and specific other non-commercial uses permitted by copyright law.

ISBN: 978-1-63750-187-0

Table of Contents

ASTHMA 1

INTRODUCTION 5

CHAPTER 1 8
   WHAT IS ASTHMA? 8
   WHAT CAUSES ASTHMA ATTACKS? 12

CHAPTER 2 19
   CAUSES OF ASTHMA 19
      Environmental Causes: 19
      Hygiene Hypothesis 21
      Genetics 22
      Medical conditions 23
      Exacerbation 25
      Actions During Pregnancy 25
      Stress 26
   CONDITIONS THAT CAUSES ASTHMA 26

CHAPTER 3 33
   TYPES OF ASTHMA 33
      Adult-Onset Asthma 33
      Allergic Asthma 35
      Asthma- Chronic Obstructive Pulmonary Disease (COPD) 38
      Exercise-Induced Bronchoconstriction (EIB) 45
      Non-Allergic Asthma 52
      Occupational Asthma 56

CHAPTER 4 61
   EXERCISE-INDUCED ASTHMA 61
      How does Exercise Induces Asthma? 61

CHAPTER 5 63

    How to Diagnose of Asthma 63

        Physical Examination 64

        Asthma Tests 65

CHAPTER 6 .... **68**

    Asthma Symptoms Treatments 68

        Reason for Asthma Treatments 69

        Treatment options 69

        The Continuing Future of Severe Asthma Treatments 74

CHAPTER 7 .... **75**

    Complications of Unmanaged Asthma 75

        How to Lessen the Threat of Complications 82

CHAPTER 8 .... **84**

    Natural Remedies for Managing Asthma 84

CHAPTER 9 .... **92**

    Natural Solution to Asthma 92

        Symptoms and Signs 92

        Natural Remedies 93

CHAPTER 10 .... **102**

    Medications for Asthma 102

Introduction

Are you aware that respiratory diseases like asthma can be managed effectively and controlled to impede the level of an asthma attack and symptoms?

Unmanaged asthma symptoms could be detrimental to your health at a time of pandemic or outbreak that attacks the respiratory system?

The symptoms of asthma often occur with periodic attacks or signs of tightness in the upper body, wheezing, difficulty breathing, and coughing.

Asthma isn't curable; nonetheless, it is controllable. For all those with severe and stubborn symptoms, a new generation of therapies - and specific treatments coming - would finally offer more relief.

Untreated asthma attacks can result in hospitalization and may even come to be fatal. It isn't a problem that needs to be neglected or handled with levity during an outbreak or pandemic like this.

Some natural treatments would be able to ease your

symptoms, decrease the amount of medication you will need to use, and generally enhance the quality of life you will ever have. These remedies work best when taken alongside your usual prescribed asthma medications.

Knowing what to do and what to avoid is crucial at a time like this. When you have severe asthma, as well as your standard medications are not providing the relief you will need, you might be curious whether there are other things you should do to handle your symptoms.

This book will teach you the simplified things you can necessarily do from home for managing, avoiding the occurrence of an asthma attack and symptoms effectively. It is an excellent resource for asthmatic patients who is conscious of the detrimental effect of unmanaged asthma symptoms during a pandemic that attacks the respiratory system.

This book is ideal for understanding;

- How to develop an asthma action plan based on the principles of assessing and treating asthma attacks,

- having full knowledge of the causes of an asthma attack and symptoms,

- natural remedies for improving the symptoms of an asthma attack, or any respiratory diseases.

- effectively managing your symptoms and prevention from the risk of exposure to more harmful respiratory diseases during an outbreak or pandemic time.

…and a lot more!

As you read further, you would be accustomed to ways of managing your asthma symptoms as well as reduce your risk of having a more deadly respiratory disease.

Chapter 1

What is Asthma?

Asthma is a chronic respiratory disease that often leads to severe episodes of symptoms. Asthma can be an incurable disease of the airways. The condition causes swelling and narrowing inside the lung, restricting air source.

The symptoms of asthma often occur with periodic attacks or signs of tightness in the upper body, wheezing, difficulty breathing, and coughing. Through the development of asthma, the airways swell and are extremely sensitive to some of the substances a person might breathe in.

When this increased level of sensitivity causes a reaction, the muscles that control the airways tighten. In doing this, they could restrict the airways even more and result in an over-production of mucus.

The group of inflammatory events in the respiratory system can result in severe symptoms of the asthma attack. Worldwide, around 250,000 people pass away every year from asthma. Asthma episodes occur when symptoms are at their peak. They could begin all of a sudden and can range between moderate to severe. In a few asthma attacks, bloating in the airways can completely prevent oxygen from getting to the lungs, which also halts it from getting into the bloodstream and planning a trip to vital organs.

This sort of asthma attack can be fatal and requires urgent hospitalization. At the beginning of the asthma attack, the airways allow enough air into the lungs, but it generally does not allow for skin tightening and leave the lungs at an easy enough rate. Skin tightening is poisonous if your body will not expel the gas, and an extended asthma attack might trigger a build-up of the gas in the lungs.

It may further decrease the amount of oxygen entering the bloodstream. People who have apparent symptoms of asthma should see a doctor. They'll provide treatments and advise on management techniques, as well as determining potential causes for asthma symptoms and how to prevent them. The doctor will also recommend medications in reducing the rate of recurrence of asthma episodes.

Asthma is a common long-term inflammatory disease of the airways of the lungs. It is characterized by adjustable and repeating symptoms, reversible airflow obstruction, and easily triggered bronchospasms. Medical indications include episodes of wheezing, coughing, chest tightness, and shortness of breathing. These might occur several times each day or several times weekly. Concerning the person, they could become worse during the night or with exercise.

Asthma is regarded as the effect of a mixture of genetic and environmental factors. Environmental factors include contact with polluting of the environment and allergens. Other potential set-offs include medications such as aspirin and beta-blockers. The analysis is usually predicated on the design of symptoms, response to therapy as time passes, and spirometers. Asthma is classified based on the frequency of symptoms, forced expiratory volume in a single second (FEV1), and top expiratory stream rate. It could also be categorized as atopic or non-atopic, where atopic identify a predisposition toward creating a type 1 hypersensitivity response.

There is no cure for asthma. Symptoms can be avoided by staying away from causes, such as allergens and irritants, and through inhaled corticosteroids. Long-Acting Beta Agonists (LABA) or ant-leukotriene agents can be utilized in addition to inhaled corticosteroids if asthma symptoms stay uncontrolled. Treatment of rapidly worsening symptoms is usually with an inhaled short-acting beta-2 agonist such as salbutamol and corticosteroids taken orally. In very severe instances, intravenous corticosteroids, magnesium sulfate, and hospitalization may be needed.

In 2015, 358 million people globally had asthma, up from 183 million in 1990. It triggered about 397,100 fatalities in 2015, the majority of which happened in the developing world. It often starts in child years. The rates of asthma have more than doubled because of the 1960s. Asthma was named early as Old Egypt. The term "asthma" is from the Greek ἄσθμα, ásthma, this means "panting."

What Causes Asthma Attacks?

Asthma is a chronic respiratory disease that often leads to severe episodes of symptoms. Asthma can be an incurable disease of the airways. The condition causes swelling and narrowing inside the lung, restricting air source.

The symptoms of asthma often occur with periodic attacks or signs of tightness in the upper body, wheezing, breathlessness, and coughing. During the development of asthma, the airways swell and are extremely sensitive to some of the substances a person might breathe in.

When this increased level of sensitivity causes a reaction, the muscles that control the airways tighten. In doing this, they could restrict the airways even more and result in an over-production of mucus.

Below are what causes asthma attack;

- Inflammation causes the airway to swell. Making the airway thin.

- The muscles around the airway tighten; this makes

the airway even slimmer.

- The small stuff going inside the airway are irritants that are trapped in the mucous. In healthy lungs, a thin film of mucus lines the airways to capture irritants such as dirt. Small hairs that gather on the airways called cilia to move backward and forwards in a whip-like movement and bring the mucous and caught contaminants up to the pharynx to be coughed up. When an asthma strike happens, too much mucus is formed. It helps it be problematic for the cilia to take it up. The already small airway now becomes clogged with mucus. This helps it become difficult, or in severe instances impossible to inhale and exhale, because air cannot flow.

They are the tiny hairs called cilia, which range within the airways. An asthma attack is when, after some time, when a person has already established just a few or no symptoms of asthma, asthma gets worse suddenly, usually because of being exposed to several triggers. When the asthma assault happens, the cells inside the airways swell because of irritation - which is the way the body attempts to safeguard itself from dangerous things, like bacteria and irritants. When the cells grow, the starting (called the lumen) in the airway gets very thin.

There are smooth muscles; (these are the type of muscles in the torso that does not contract voluntarily, like the ones in the arm) across the bronchi and bronchioles start to spasm or contract, making the opening in the airway even narrower. That is called a ***bronchospasm.***

In the lining of the airways are glands called, ***submucosal glands***, and above them, near the beginning of the airway are cells called ***goblet cells*** - because they're shaped similar to a goblet, which looks like a cup. The submucosal glands and the goblet cells produce mucus that helps protect the inner of the airways. The mucus in the airways of healthy lungs is a thin film that traps irritants such as dirt contaminants and pollen, so they don't harm the airways and keep them from getting into the environment sacs (alveoli).

You will find tiny hairs lining the airway called ***cilia***. The cilia influxes backward and forwards just like little whips, and help drive the mucus and the stuck particles in the airways to the "pharynx. Following that, the mucous, the captured particles from the low airways can be coughed up (*sputum*).

During an asthma strike, the submucosal glands and the goblet cells start making a lot more mucus than usual, and the mucus is also thicker than usual; this helps it become challenging for the cilia to do their job, and bring the mucus up from the airways. So, there is too much mucus being made, rather than enough being raised by the cilia. The airways are already also slim to inhale appropriately because of the tissue swelling triggered by swelling and the constriction triggered by the bronchospasms. Therefore the extra mucus blocks the airway even more; this makes respiration very hard. In fatal asthma episodes, the airways may become so constricted and connected with mucus that no air can pass through effortlessly.

You can find other signs of breathing difficulty as in an asthma attack, which is essential to learn, and knowing them can help tell if a person who cannot talk is having difficulty in breathing. People who might not have the ability to let someone know they are experiencing difficulty in breathing include infants and small children.

- ***Intercostal retractions***

The skin between your ribs appears 'sucked in' as the intercostal muscles (located between your bones) deal more than usual. This happens to help your body ingest more air due to difficulty in deep breathing. Intercostal retractions are an indicator of inhaling and exhaling stress and a possible indication of worsening asthma or an asthma assault.

A number of the other signals of asthma include:

- ***Chest and throat retractions***, which cause muscles within the upper body and throat not usually used too much during respiration to start contracting as they try to help to ingest more air. Retractions are the way the body attempts to get enough air because of the issue in deep breathing generally because of the asthma strike. These retractions cause your skin of the upper body wall, your skin of the throat, and or the breastbone (sternum) to go in when inhaling and exhaling. There will vary types of retractions that relax when muscles start contracting, which depends on how much difficulty one is having breathing during an attack.

- *Nose flaring*: is when the starting of the nostrils gets bigger than usual during respiration. It is a sign a person is having difficulty in deep breathing.

- *Blue lip area and fingertips*: air, which is within the environment we breathe, is why the bloodstream is having a red colorization. Blood without air has a blue color. Air enters your body through the environment sacs **(alveoli),** which are at the end of the airways. During an asthma attack, it is problematic for your body to get enough oxygen since it is difficult to get enough air, which certainly reduces red blood (blood with oxygen in it) and more blue blood (blood without oxygen in it). The blue color of the lips and under the fingernails is due to the blue blood, which may be seen in the tiny arteries under your skin. More areas of the body start turning blue, and the body goes without oxygen. When areas of the body become blue because of insufficient oxygen, it is named *cyanosis.*

Chapter 2
Causes of Asthma

Asthma is the effect of a combination of organic and incompletely understood environmental and genetic relationships, which influences both its severity and its responsiveness to treatment. It is thought that the recently increased rates of asthma are credited to changing epigenetics (heritable factors apart from those related to the DNA series) and a changing living environment. Onset before age 12 is more likely credited to hereditary influence, while onset after age 12 is more likely credited to environmental impact.

Environmental Causes:

Many environmental factors have been associated with asthma's development and exacerbation, including allergens, polluting of the environment, and other environmental chemicals. Smoking during pregnancy and after delivery is associated with a more significant threat of asthma-like symptoms. Low quality of air from factors such as traffic pollution or high ozone levels has been associated with both asthma development and increased asthma severity. Over fifty percent (50%) of situations in children in America occur in areas with quality of air below EPA standards. Low quality of air is more prevalent in low-income and minority communities.

Contact with indoor volatile organic substances may be considered a result of asthma; formaldehyde exposure has a positive association. Also, phthalates types of PVC are associated with asthma in both children and adults. While contact with pesticides can bring about the development of asthma, a reason and a productive relationship have yet been found.

There can be an association between acetaminophen (paracetamol) use and asthma. A lot of the evidence will not, however, support a causal role. A 2014 review discovered that the association disappeared when respiratory infections were considered. Use by a mom during pregnancy is also associated with an elevated risk of mental stress during pregnancy.

Asthma is associated with contact with indoor allergens. Common indoor allergens include dust mites, cockroaches, animal dander (fragments of fur or feathers), and mold. Attempts to diminish dust mites are inadequate on symptoms in the sensitized subject matter. Certain viral respiratory system infections, such as respiratory system syncytial virus and rhinovirus, may boost the risk of growing asthma when ingested by small children.

Hygiene Hypothesis

The hygiene hypothesis attempts to clarify the increased rates of asthma worldwide as a primary and unintended consequence of reduced exposure, during childhood, to non-pathogenic bacteria and viruses. It's been proposed that the reduced contact with bacterial infections is due, partly, to increased cleanliness and reduced family size in modern societies. Contact with bacterial endotoxin in early years as a child may avoid the development of asthma, but exposure at a mature age group may provoke broncho-constriction. Proof supporting the cleanliness hypothesis includes lower rates of asthma on farms and in households with domestic pets.

The use of antibiotics in early life has been from the development of asthma. Also, delivery via cesarean section is associated with an elevated risk (estimated at 20-80%) of asthma. This increased risk is related to having less healthy bacterial colonization that the newborn could have acquired from passing through the delivery canal. There's a link between asthma and the amount of affluence which might be related to the hygiene hypothesis as less affluent individuals frequently have more contact with bacterial infections.

Genetics

Genealogy is a risk factor for asthma, with numerous genes being implicated. If one identical twin is affected, the likelihood of the other getting the disease is approximately 25%. At the end of 2005, 25 genes have been associated with asthma in six or even more separate populations, including GSTM1, IL10, CTLA-4, SPINK5, LTC4S, IL4R, and ADAM33, amongst others. Several genes are related to disease fighting capability or modulating inflammation. Even among this set of genes backed by highly replicated studies, results never have been constant among all populations examined. In 2006, over 100 genes were associated with asthma in single genetic association research alone; presently, more is found.

Some hereditary variants may only cause asthma when they are related to specific environmental exposures. A functional examination is sole nucleotide polymorphism contact with endotoxin (a bacterial product). Endotoxin exposure will come from several ecological resources, including tobacco cigarettes, canines, and farms. The risk of asthma then depends on both someone's genetics and the amount of endotoxin exposure.

Medical conditions

A triad of atopic eczema, allergic rhinitis, and asthma is

named *atopy*. The most potent risk factor for growing asthma is a brief history of atopic disease, with asthma occurring at a much higher rate in those people who have either eczema or hay fever. Asthma is associated with eosinophilic granulomatosis with polyangiitis (formerly known as Churg-Strauss symptoms), autoimmune disease, and vasculitis. People with certain types of urticaria could also experience the symptoms of asthma.

There's a correlation between obesity and the chance of asthma, with both having increased lately. Several factors may be at play, including reduced respiratory function due to a buildup of fat and the fact that a disposed of tissue leads to a pro-inflammatory state.

Beta-blocker medications such as propranolol can cause asthma in those who find themselves vulnerable. Cardio selective beta-blockers, however, show up safe in people that have a slight or moderate disease. Other medications that can cause problems in asthmatics are angiotensin-converting enzyme inhibitors, aspirin, and NSAIDs. The use of acidity suppressing drug (proton pump inhibitors and H2 blockers) during pregnancy is associated with an elevated threat of asthma in the child.

Exacerbation

A lot of people will have steady asthma for weeks and then suddenly develop a bout of acute asthma. Different individuals respond to various factors in various ways. Most individuals can form severe exacerbations from lots of triggering brokers.

Home factors that can result in worsening of asthma include dirt, pet dander (especially kitty and dog locks), cockroach allergens, and mildew. Perfumes are a common reason behind severe attacks in women and children. Both viral and bacterial attacks of the top respiratory system can worsen the condition. Psychological stress may worsen symptoms - it is thought that stress alters the disease fighting capability and thus escalates the airway inflammatory response to allergens and irritants.

Actions During Pregnancy

If a female smokes a cigarette or illicit substances while pregnant, an unborn child might grow less in the womb, experience problems during labor and delivery, and also have a minimal birth weight.

These newborns might become more susceptible to medical issues, including asthma.

Stress

Individuals who undergo stress have higher asthma rates. Raises in asthma-related behaviors during difficult times, such as smoking, may reduce these increased rates.

Psychological responses, such as grief, might trigger asthma attacks.

Conditions that Causes Asthma

A doctor could use a stethoscope to pay attention to panting noises in someone's lungs. Wheezing is an indicator of asthma.

- *Wheezing/Panting*

Wheezing sounds noticed with a stethoscope. Signs or

symptoms in medication will be the way a condition affects someone's body. Sometimes the signs or symptoms of asthma may be minor, which will not bother the individual too much. At other times, they might be severe, which might make the individual feel very ill.

Don't assume all persons with asthma has all the signs or symptoms of asthma regularly. A person may involve some signs or symptoms during one asthma assault and also have different symptoms during another asthma strike. Some individuals with asthma may have extended periods between asthma episodes, where they show no symptoms and experience no symptoms of asthma. In contrast, some may show some or all the signs or symptoms every day, which are more severe during an assault. It also depends on which kind of asthma one has and if they have a slight, moderate, or severe case.

There are also many people with asthma who might have signs or symptoms during such as exercise-induced asthma, where the activity triggers the symptoms. For a few, the signs or symptoms of asthma may be brought on or compounded (exacerbated) when they have viral respiratory system infections, usually the type caused by human being rhinoviruses.

Early indicators of the asthma attack are physical changes in health a person with asthma has before they have the seizure. By knowing the first indicators, a person might be able to do something to avoid having an asthma strike or if indeed, they do have one, to keep it from getting worse.

The early indicators of asthma can include:

- Coughing a lot, especially during the night.

- You are dropping your breath quickly.

- **Shortness of breathing:** this is whenever a person cannot take a breath, which means they cannot fill up their lungs completely with air. They might be in a position to make brief, shallow breaths that will give their lungs enough air. Whenever a person has shortness of breath, they may likewise have chest tightness.

Getting exhausted quickly during exercise and sense

weak and wheezing or hacking and coughing after use. Since the symptoms of a cold or allergies arriving on like sneezing, a runny or stuffed up nose area, hacking and coughing, sore throat, and headache.

- *Triggers*

These are a few things that could make someone's asthma worse and can result in an asthma assault.

A cause factor or result, in brief, is something that triggers the signs of a condition to start in someone who already has that condition. Some common set-offs for asthma are:

- *Tobacco smoke from cigarettes:* a person doesn't need to smoke cigarettes themselves, smoke from cigarettes can cause an asthma strike. Smoke from cigarettes is the remains of burning up a cigarette, cigar, or tube that another person is smoking or the smoke from cigarettes that they exhale.

- *Pets:* animals produce chemicals called proteins that trigger allergies; people can be hypersensitive to them. These things that trigger allergies can become irritants and make someone's asthma worse and result in an asthma assault. The proteins are in the pet's dander, which is the dead flakes of pores and skin that pets (and folks) shed. Also, they are in their urine, faeces, saliva, and sebum, which is manufactured by glands in the skin called sebaceous glands. Sebum is why hair epidermis is oily. When dander, urine, faeces, saliva, and sebum dry up, their proteins may become airborne and breathed in. A number of the types of household pets' people can be sensitive to are canines, pet cats, gerbils, hamsters, guinea pigs, and family pet birds.

- *Bugs:* different kinds of pests that might be found in homes may cause asthma attacks. They could result in asthma symptoms just as house animals; the proteins they provide are things that trigger allergies and are airborne. A number of the more common insects which may cause asthma are dirt mites, cockroaches, and also bedbugs and fleas. Many other varieties that may infest a home may serve as a way to obtain allergens such as Pharaoh ants.

- ***Fungi spores (mildew)***: fungi reproduce by releasing spores into the air; if the spores land in the right place, the growth of a new fungi starts. Sucking in these spores can result in asthma. Among the most typical types of fungi spores within both outdoors and outside conditions are from a species (genus) known aspergillus.

Strong feelings such as anger, stress, and even laughter, may get asthma symptoms worse.

Outdoor polluting of the environment comes from many sources such as car and truck fumes in regions of heavy traffic and chemicals in the air close to factories and refineries.

- *Weather:* changes in the elements of weather can cause an asthma strike. Changes in the wind, heat can result in an attack, not only chilly air. If a person goes from being outside in the cool into a warm house, the unexpected change can result in bronchospasm. Sudden changes in moisture also play a serious role.

The ultimate way to deal with asthma triggers is to learn what they are and prevent them when possible, and if not avoided, they can change one's behavior to cope with them. For example, operating on the frosty winter day right up to the doorstep of the warm house and heading immediately inside, the unexpected temperature change can cause an assault and could be prevented.

Generally, but especially with a condition, for such asthma, it's essential to understand one's environment and what's in it, both indoors and outdoors. Frequently, Asthma is induced by things that trigger allergies. One big way to get items that trigger allergies is the carpet. Replacing it with a tiled floor decreases the possibility of making a suitable environment for the things that trigger allergies, which is more straightforward to completely clean and disinfect.

Chapter 3

Types of Asthma

Adult-Onset Asthma

Some individuals don't show signs of experiencing asthma until they are adults. That is known as **adult-onset asthma.**

What can cause adult-onset asthma? There are numerous possible factors.

Sometimes, people can ignore their asthma causes for years. If they are later subject to that cause as a grown-up adult, it may bring on asthma symptoms. For instance, they may move around with a roommate that has a family pet, or they could work around certain chemical substance fumes for the very first time.

Other times, a viral infection can unmask their asthma symptoms. For instance, they may come with a top respiratory disease leading to coughing that sticks around for weeks.

Symptoms:

The most frequent signs of asthma are:

- Coughing, especially during the night, during exercise or when laughing.

- Difficulty breathing.

- Chest tightness.

- Shortness of breath.

- Wheezing.

Diagnosis:

An allergist can see whether you have *adult-onset asthma* by doing checks that will assist in making a diagnosis.

Treatment and Management:

It could be frustrating to find as a grown-up that you will now be facing a chronic condition like asthma. Nonetheless, it doesn't have to set you back.

The trick to successfully managing your asthma is to use an allergist. Collectively, you can identify your set-offs and create a plan to prevent them. Your allergist can also recommend quick-relief and long-term control medications.

Life's too brief to have a problem with asthma. If you discover an allergist, who could work with you to produce a plan and stay with it, there's no reason asthma must change anything about how exactly you live your daily life.

Allergic Asthma

There is usually a tie between allergies and asthma.

Not everyone that has allergy has asthma, rather than everyone with asthma has allergies. But things that trigger allergies such as pollen, dirt, and pet dander can result in asthma symptoms and asthma episodes in people.

Symptoms:

The most frequent signs of this type of asthma are:

- Coughing, especially during the night, during exercise or when laughing.

- Difficulty breathing.

- Tightness in the chest.

- Shortness of breath.

- Wheezing.

- Diagnosis.

Allergic asthma can be intensified by factors that cause non-allergic asthma, such as viral respiratory system infections, exercise, irritants in the air, stress, drugs and certain food chemicals, and climate. Whatever causes your symptoms, your allergist is most beneficially outfitted to diagnose asthma, determine its trigger factors and whether they are caused by allergies, and offer the best plan for your treatment. An allergist can see whether you have allergic asthma by doing tests that will assist in making a diagnosis.

Treatment and Management:

Allergists are specially trained to help you manage your asthma and allergy symptoms to be able to live the life span you want - without limits.

By taking a family group background and conducting screening through pores and skin or blood testing, an allergist could work with you to recognize the allergens that are triggering your asthma.

Your allergist can also help you create and intend to manage your trouble. This plan ranges from quick-relief and long-term asthma controlling medications, as well as methods for staying away from triggers such as:

- Pollen from turf, trees, and shrubs, and weeds.

- Pet dander.

- Dust mites.

- Mold

Your allergist can also help you treat the underlying allergy that is triggering your asthma. One treatment is *allergy immunotherapy*, which is a preventive treatment that helps the body become less delicate to specific things that trigger allergies. It's accomplished by two medications: *allergy shots and sublingual tablets* that dissolve under the tongue. Make sure to discuss this and other treatment plans with your allergist.

Asthma- Chronic Obstructive Pulmonary Disease (COPD)

Asthma is known to be severe when it's challenging to take care of and manage the symptoms.

Chronic Obstructive Pulmonary Disease (COPD) is an assortment of lung diseases that cause difficulty in breathing and obstruct airflow. This band of disease ranges from refractory (severe) asthma, emphysema, and chronic bronchitis.

A lot of people with asthma won't develop COPD, and many people who have COPD don't have asthma. However, it's possible to have both. Asthma-COPD overlap symptoms (ACOS) occur when someone has both of these diseases simultaneously.

Symptoms:

Indicators of ACOS include:

- Difficulty breathing.
- Wheezing.
- Frequent coughing.
- Tightness in the chest.
- Excess phlegm.
- Feeling tired.
- Low physical tolerance for exercise.
- Shortness of breath during program activities.

Although symptoms might not continually be severe, ACOS is severe and can be deadly. In 2014, chronic lower respiratory diseases - mainly COPD - were the 3rd leading reason behind death in the U.S., based on the Centers for Disease Control and Prevention. About 3,500 people die of asthma every year, almost half of whom are age 65 or older.

People who have asthma might not realize there is also

COPD. Sometimes COPD isn't diagnosed until it's in the "moderate" stage, indicating they may be experiencing regular shortness of breathing, hacking and coughing, and heavier-than-normal mucus. Mis-diagnosis may appear because the symptoms of COPD mimic those of asthma.

Triggers:

Asthma causes often include allergens, such as *pollen, dirt mites, cockroaches, molds, and pet dander*. Things that trigger allergies can make COPD symptoms worse. And if remaining untreated, allergy symptoms and asthma can raise the chances for COPD in individuals. But COPD is not similar to asthma, and COPD is not triggered by allergy symptoms or asthma. COPD is an assortment of lung diseases. However, COPD can be derived from long-term contact with a few of the same environmental risk factors - often in workplaces - which can also cause occupational asthma.

Smoking is the foremost risk factor for developing COPD. Smoking is an unhealthy aggravation to all or any respiratory problems. It could decrease your life span and hinder your treatment solution. The main thing you can do for your wellbeing is to avoid smoking.

Diagnosis:

When someone has ACOS, it's possible to mistake asthma for COPD or vice versa and neglect to recognize the existence of both conditions. When you have either severe asthma or COPD, you should demand further testing to discover if you have ACOS. When both of these diseases overlap, both disorders have to be treated.

A diagnosis of severe asthma means that the symptoms of your asthma aren't responding well to medications typically used to control asthma, such as inhaled corticosteroids. You'll need special treatment and medication to attempt to improve lung function and manage symptoms. It's important to consider other ailments at this time to find out if other factors are adding to the medical diagnosis of severe asthma.

COPD is diagnosed most regularly among specific kind of people:

- People between age groups of 50 and 74.

- Current and previous smokers.

- People with a history of severe asthma.

- People who have long-term exposure airborne irritants, including commercial chemicals and cigarette smoke.

- People with a family background of COPD

While COPD is regarded as an ailment most regularly diagnosed in older white men, a 2013 report by the American Lung Association discovered that women are 37% much more likely than men to have the disease and constitute over fifty percent of the COPD deaths in the U.S.

Early diagnosis and treatment can transform the span of the syndrome and slow down its progression. An allergist can diagnose COPD and other conditions, such as asthma, by requesting your health background. Your allergist will also offer you a physical examination that can include a quick inhaling and exhaling test, known as spirometry, which will measure how much air your lungs can take and exactly how quickly air flows in and out.

Your allergist also may suggest an upper-body CT check and an upper body X-ray. After identifying the stage of your COPD as well as your asthma, which ranges from light to severe, your allergist will review treatment plans with you and discuss changes in lifestyle and cure intend to ensure you are feeling better and improve lung function.

Treatment and Management:

COPD is progressive; this means it gets worse as time passes. Asthma is a reversible condition when the right treatment is received at the right time, which makes early treatment important, mainly when ACOS occurs.

When you have any indicators of COPD, you should see an allergist. The sooner you get treatment, the better. Your allergist is specially trained to help you manage the chronic conditions of asthma, COPD, or ACOS. It's especially important to get your allergist to control symptoms and get the best treatment feasible for your particular needs.

Treating ACOS isn't a one-size-fits-all approach. Each patient receives a personalized treatment solution. Treatment can include medication to lessen symptoms, supplemental air, and pulmonary (lung) treatment. It might take some time to recognize which drugs work right for you. Changes in lifestyle, such as *exercise, breathing techniques, and avoidance of air pollutants at home and work, can also be recommended.* For smokers, the most crucial part of treatment is *quitting the utilization of tobacco.*

Because respiratory health problems like the flu can cause severe problems in people who have ACOS, you should get an annual flu vaccine. A pneumococcal pneumonia vaccine is also suggested.

The sooner you contact an allergist, the better. There is no remedy for ACOS, and the first diagnosis of the syndrome can enhance the general health of your lungs. When several illnesses impact your respiration or if you have ACOS, your allergist can help you manage your symptoms and maximize your lung function. Don't wait to find an allergist. Act fast now to boost your wellbeing and the grade of your life.

Exercise-Induced Bronchoconstriction (EIB)

Exercise-induced Bronchoconstriction, or EIB, is the most well-liked term for that which was known for a long time as *Exercise-induced Asthma*. Symptoms develop when airways become narrow because of exercise. As much as 90 percent of individuals with asthma likewise have EIB; however, not everyone with EIB has asthma. Many elite and world-class athletes have EIB - including Olympic medal winners in sports like cross-country skiing, figure skating, and ice hockey. EIB didn't hold them back, and it shouldn't hold you back either.

An allergist will customize a cure plan which allows you to make contact with the exercise you like and feel better while carrying it out.

Symptoms:

EIB is caused by the increased loss of heat, drinking

water, or both from the airways during exercise when quickly sucking in air that is drier than what is already in the torso. Symptoms typically show up within minutes once you start working out and could continue for 10mins to quarter-hour once you finish your workout. Anyone can experience these symptoms (especially somebody who has gone out of shape), but with EIB, these are more serious. Wheezing in children after exercise is usually the first symptom of asthma.

Common symptoms of EIB include:

- Shortness of breathing or wheezing

- Decreased endurance.

- Tightness in the chest.

- Cough.

- Upset stomach.

- Sore throat

EIB set offs include airborne irritants related to specific sports activities. Examples are:

- Chorine when swimming.

- Pollution while working or cycling.

- Cold, dried out air while snow skating or taking part in hockey.

- Air temperatures during hot yoga exercise.

If you are training in a fitness center, perfume, cleaners, color, and new equipment or carpet may become a trigger.

Although it was thought for a long time that breathing cold air makes EIB worse, further studies indicate that the dryness of the environment, as opposed to the temperature, is much more likely the trigger. Cold air typically contains less moisture than heated air, and quick breathing dry air dehydrates the bronchial tubes, leading to these to narrow and restrict airflow.

The sports and activities that are likely to cause EIB symptoms to require continuous activity are done in winter. Included in these are soccer, golf ball, long-distance running, glaciers hockey, snow skating, and cross-country snowboarding.

The actions that are least more likely to cause EIB medical indications include walking, hiking, and recreational biking, or sports requiring only short bursts of activity. Included in these are volleyball, gymnastics, football, wrestling, golf, going swimming, soccer, and short-distance monitor and field sports. Some swimming events can demand continuous activity; however, the warmth and humidity from the water make it easier for individuals with EIB to breathe.

Diagnosis:

Have you got EIB? Sometimes this is difficult for sports athletes to learn. Everyone has already established a problem completing good work sometimes, and athletes don't often think of EIB or asthma as the reason. An allergist can determine whether your symptoms are exercise-induced only, or a reaction to things that trigger allergies or irritants in the air, or are a sign of underlying asthma.

Within an examination, your allergist will need a brief history (such as requesting information about any loved ones with asthma or other profound breathing difficulties). Additionally, you may be asked specific information regarding your exercise, including where and exactly how often you exercise. Your allergist will also consider other conditions, such as upper-airway problems, that may likely be involved in your issues with exercise.

To check on how exercise impacts your respiration, your allergist may measure your deep breathing before, after, and during operation on a treadmill machine or ride on a fitness bike. During the test, you will inhale and exhale into a pipe that connects to a spirometer, a tool that measures the quantity of air being inhaled and exhaled.

In some instances, environmental factors may contribute to EIB. Skaters and hockey players can be suffering from a mixture of cold, dried out the air in glaciers rinks and contaminants from ice-resurfacing machines. EIB in distance joggers has been associated with working out in high-allergen and high-ozone conditions. Furthermore, indoor air with high degrees of trichloramine, a chemical substance found in pool chlorination, has been associated with asthma and EIB in swimmers.

Treatment and Management:

Two types of medications used to take care of asthma are also used to avoid and treat EIB symptoms. They're usually made via an *inhaler*, while some can be purchased in tablet form:

- *Short-acting inhaled beta2-agonists* (bronchodilators) stop signs immediately. They might be used 15 to 30 minutes before strenuous exercises and generally prevent symptoms for just 2 to 4 hours. These medications are effective in dealing with or avoiding EIB symptoms, so if symptoms do not improve, let your allergist know.

- *Long-term control asthma medicines;* are taken daily to prevent symptoms and attacks.

- *Inhaled corticosteroids;* are the most recommended long-term asthma medications. They help reduce the narrowing and irritation of the bronchial pipes. It might take two to a month before these drugs reach their maximum impact.

- *Long-acting inhaled beta2-agonists (bronchodilators);* Used 30 to 60 minutes before exercise; these medications assist in preventing symptoms for 10 to 12 hours. They must be used only one time within 12 hours, plus they should be used only in mixture with an inhaled corticosteroid.

- *Montelukast, a leukotriene receptor inhibitor,* is also approved for treating *Exercise-induced Asthma symptoms*. It can be used once daily; this medication helps in preventing symptoms that accompany exercise.

Elite sports athletes should talk with the regulating bodies of their sport about the medicines they may be allowed to use to relieve their EIB or asthma symptoms. Another source is the Prohibited List, released by the World Anti-Doping Company. Some medications (including beta2-alpha) are believed to be performance-enhancing drugs and can't be utilized by athletes in competition unless a therapeutic use exemption is granted for medical needs. Your allergist will help you answer questions about your medications.

Other recommendations for relieving symptoms of EIB include:

- Warm-up with easy exercises for approximately 15 minutes before you begin a more intense workout.

- Cover the mouth area and nose with a scarf or nose and mouth mask when you exercise in winter.

- Make an effort to breathe through your nasal area during exercise. It would help warm the environment that switches into your lungs.

- Avoid triggers by making changes to your workout routine.

See an allergist for prescription medications, which might be far better than over-the-counter treatments.

Non-Allergic Asthma

Does your asthma symptoms flare up in extreme weather

condition, either in the heat of summer or the chill of winter? When you get unwell, does it often lead to an asthma assault? Does stress bring about breathing problems?

If this is the case, you may be experiencing non-allergic asthma.

Symptoms:

The most frequent signs of asthma are:

- Coughing, especially during the night, during exercise or when laughing.

- Difficulty breathing.

- Tightness in the chest.

- Shortness of breath.

- Wheezing.

Triggers:

As the name implies, non-allergic asthma is triggered by

factors different from allergens. These ranges from;

- Viral respiratory system infections.

- Exercise.

- Irritants in the air.

- Stress.

- Drugs and food additives.

- Weather conditions.

Diagnosis:

You may wonder why you need to visit an allergist for non-allergic asthma. Asthma can be activated by many factors, even in the same person. But allergy symptoms are the most typical of these causes. Therefore, everyone with asthma or suspected asthma should be examined by an allergist to see whether this typical result is playing a job in his/her breathing problems.

Allergists are specially trained to help you manage your allergy symptoms and asthma, and that means you can live the life span you want. An allergist can see whether you have non-allergic asthma by doing examinations that will assist in making a diagnosis.

Treatment and Management:

When you can't tie up your asthma to a particular allergen, such as dog fur or house dirt, it could be harder to recognize your set-offs. That's why it's essential to consult an allergist - to access the leading cause of your asthma and create a solution to manage it.

Allergists can prescribe quick-relief and long-term control medicines. They are also able to make you recognize and steer clear of triggers and make an idea for avoiding asthma attacks.

Occupational Asthma

Overview

People with this problem usually come around chemical substance fumes, dirt, or other irritants in the air. If you've been identified as having asthma that has another cause, it could be worsened by airborne irritants at work. When you have asthma and believe that your place of work is leading to or worsening your symptoms, your allergist will help you manage your disease.

Is your asthma triggered by your work?

This question may be challenging to answer. You'll need to solve other issues first, including:

- Does your asthma start when you transformed jobs?

- Will your asthma improve if you are away from your job?

- Do chemicals and other conditions make it difficult to breathe?

Proof of Occupational Asthma:

The Occupational Safety and Health Academy (OSHA) reports an estimated 11 million employees in an array of industries and occupations in America to face at least one of the more than 250 substances known or thought to cause or exacerbate occupational asthma. Occupational factors are associated with up to 15% of disabling asthma cases. Triggers can include chemicals found in manufacturing; paints; cleaning products; dust from wood, grain and flour; latex gloves; certain molds; animals; and insects. Factors that boost the risk for developing occupational asthma include existing allergies or asthma, a group history of allergies or asthma, and using tobacco.

Based on the Countrywide Institutes of Health, the next workers are in increased threat of developing occupational asthma:

- Bakers.

- Detergent manufacturers.

- Drug manufacturers.

- Farmers.

- Grain elevator workers.

- Laboratory employees (especially those dealing with laboratory pets).

- Metalworkers.

- Millers.

- Plastics workers.

- Woodworkers

Identifying whether your asthma is work-related will demand an intensive physical examination. Expect your allergist to:

- ✓ Take a health background that reveals whether any of your loved ones have allergies, asthma, or other allergic diseases, such as eczema.

- ✓ Request you to describe your present and past jobs and consider whether they seem related to your asthma. You ought to be able to clarify your task and job conditions, such as contact with fumes, gases, smoke, irritants, chemicals, and potential allergens. It's also advisable to discuss environmental conditions, such as heat, cold or dryness, as well as any manufacturing or processing conditions that you are exposed to.

- ✓ Ask you about your symptoms - how often they happen and what appears to trigger them.

- ✓ Perform lung function lab tests, such as spirometry, an instant and painless test that steps airflow.

- ✓ Additionally, your allergist may perform skin tests and order chest X-rays and blood tests. If indicated, aerosol problem studies may be considered.

It might be helpful that you should obtain information on your occupational exposures from your project's supervisor, who can provide you OSHA safety guide that describes possible work-related problems. Review and offer to your allergist the Materials Safety Data Sheet (MSDS) for every chemical substance to which you're exposed to at work.

Controlling Occupational Asthma

The prevention and treatment of occupational asthma require environmental interventions, including education on behavioral changes to avoid asthma causes, along with medication therapies and careful medical follow-up. Whether you can avoid things that cause or aggravate your asthma at the job depends on where you work and what you do there. If you believe that your asthma is triggered by conditions at work, or if it worsens at work, speak to your allergist, who may recommend actions you can take to distance yourself from set offs or reduce their impact.

Chapter 4

Exercise-induced Asthma

What is Exercise-induced Asthma?

Like it sounds, Exercise-induced Asthma is asthma that is triggered by vigorous or long-term exercise. A lot of people with persistent asthma experience the symptoms of asthma during exercise. However, there are numerous people without chronic asthma who develop symptoms only during training.

How does Exercise Induces Asthma?

During normal deep breathing, the environment we ingest is first warmed and moistened by the nose passages. Because people tend to inhale through their mouths when they exercise, these are inhaling colder and drier air.

In exercise-induced asthma, the muscle bands throughout the airways are delicate to these changes in temperature and humidity and respond by contracting, which narrow the airway, which leads to symptoms of exercise-induced Asthma, such as:

- Coughing with asthma.

- Tightening of the chest.

- Wheezing.

- Unusual fatigue while exercising.

- Shortness of breathing when exercising

The symptoms of Exercise-induced Asthma generally start within 5 to 20 minutes following the start of exercise, or 5 to 10 minutes after a short activity has stopped. If you're experiencing these symptoms with practice, inform your doctor.

Chapter 5

How to Diagnose of Asthma

Asthma diagnosis: *Health background, observations throughout a physical examination,* and *results from breathing tests.*

A doctor will administer these assessments and determine the amount of asthma's slight, intermittent, moderate, or severe symptoms in people who show indicators of the problem, as well as identifying the sort.

A detailed genealogy of asthma allergies can help a health care provider make a precise diagnosis. A personal history of allergy symptoms is also important to say, as many talks about systems with asthma boost the risk.

Keep a record of any potential causes of asthma symptoms to help guide treatment, including information about any potential irritants at work.

Make sure to identify any health issues that can hinder asthma management, such as:

- A runny nose.

- Sinus infections.

- Acid reflux.

- Psychological stress.

- Sleep apnea.

Small children who develop asthma symptoms before the age of 5 years think it is more challenging to receive a definite diagnosis. Doctors might confuse asthma symptoms with those of other youth conditions.

If children experience wheezing episodes during colds or respiratory system infections in early life, they will probably develop asthma after six years.

Physical Examination

A physical examination will generally concentrate on the upper respiratory system, chest, and pores and skin. A health care provider will pay attention to indications of wheezing, or a high-pitched whistle on deep breathing out, in the lungs throughout a breath utilizing a stethoscope. Wheezing is an integral indication of both an obstructed airway and asthma.

Doctors will also look for a runny nasal area, swollen nose passages, and soft growths within the nasal area and look for epidermis conditions, including eczema and hives. They are painful conditions that connect to asthma and suggest heightened immune system activity that may be leading to any wheezing.

People who have asthma do not necessarily show physical symptoms, which is possible to have asthma without presenting any physical maladies during an evaluation.

Asthma Tests

Lung function tests are another element of an asthma diagnosis. They measure how much air a person inhales and exhales and the velocity with which an individual can expel air from the lungs.

- A spirometry test can offer a sign of lung function.

- Spirometry can help evaluate lung function.

- *Spirometry* is a non-invasive test that will require deep breaths and forceful exhalation into a hose. The hose links to a machine called a spirometer that presents two vital measurements:

- *Forced Essential Capacity* (FVC), or the utmost amount of air an individual can breathe in and out

- *Pressured Expiratory Volume* (FEV-1), the maximum amount of air an individual can exhale in a single second

- The doctor then compares these measurements against what would be reasonable for someone of the same age. Frequencies below standard shows obstructed airways and possible asthma.

A doctor will most likely administer a bronchodilator medication to open up air passages before re-testing with the spirometer to verify the analysis if results improve after using the drug, the risk of the asthma diagnosis increases.

Children under five years are challenging to check using spirometry, and asthma diagnoses will rely mainly on symptoms, medical histories, and other areas of the physical examination process.

In youngsters, doctors commonly prescribe asthma medicines for four to six weeks to gauge the physical response.

Chapter 6
Asthma Symptoms Treatments

Asthma is an illness where the airways distend and tighten, making it hard trying to catch your breath. *Medical indications include:*

- Wheezing,

- shortness of breath,

- chest tightness.

Symptoms could be worse in a few people and less in others. You may just have symptoms at times - like when you exercise. Or you might have frequent asthma attacks that affect yourself.

Asthma isn't curable; nonetheless, it is controllable. Today's treatments are far better than previously at preventing asthma attacks - with stopping symptoms if indeed they do start. Yet 5 to 10 percent of people who have asthma don't react to standard treatments like inhaled corticosteroids.

For all those with severe and stubborn symptoms, a new generation of therapies - and specific treatments coming - would finally offer some relief.

Reason for Asthma Treatments

Asthma treatment involves a three-part strategy:

- provide long-term control medications to avoid symptoms before they start,

- quick-relief medications to prevent asthma attacks,

- avoiding triggers to lessen the number of seizures.

To regulate severe asthma, you may want to have higher doses of medications or use several drugs. You, as well as your doctor, can create an asthma action, intend to personalize your treatment strategy predicated on your symptoms and disease severity.

Treatment options

The primary treatment for severe asthma is long-term control medications that assist in preventing asthma symptoms. *Included in these are:*

- *inhaled corticosteroids,*

- *inhaled long-acting beta-agonists,*

- *inhaled long-acting anticholinergics,*

- *leukotriene modifiers,*

- *cromolyn sodium (Intal),*

- *theophylline (Theochron),*

- *oral corticosteroids.*

You can take quick-relief medications when you have an asthma attack to alleviate symptoms. Included in these are:

- inhaled short-acting beta-agonists,

- inhaled short-acting anticholinergics,

- a combined mix of an inhaled short-acting anticholinergic and inhaled short-acting beta-agonist.

Several newer treatments have made severe asthma better

to control.

Biologics

Biologic drugs use your disease-fighting capability to take care of asthma. They block the experience of disease-fighting capability chemicals that produce your airways distend. These drugs can prevent you from getting asthma attacks and make the attacks reduced.

Four monoclonal antibodies are approved to take care of severe asthma:

- *reslizumab (Cinqair),*
- *mepolizumab (Nucala),*
- *omalizumab (Xolair),*
- *benralizumab (Fasenra).*

Omalizumab treats severe asthma that's triggered by allergies. **Mepolizumab, reslizumab,** and **benralizumab**

treat severe asthma, which is the effect of a kind of white blood cell named an eosinophil (eosinophilic asthma). You consider these drugs by injection or via an IV right into a vein. New monoclonal antibodies such as *tezepelumab* are under investigation.

Tiotropium (Spiriva)

This inhaled medication has been used to take care of chronic obstructive pulmonary disease (COPD) for more than a decade. In 2015, the FDA also approved it for treating asthma. Studies also show that *tiotropium* improves asthma control when putting into high doses of inhaled corticosteroids plus short-acting beta-agonists.

Leukotriene modifiers

This band of asthma drugs works by blocking the action of *leukotriene*. This chemical tightens and narrows your airways during an allergy-induced asthma attack.

Three leukotriene modifiers are approved to take care of

asthma:

- *montelukast (Singulair),*
- *zafirlukast (Accolate),*
- *zileuton (Zyflo),*

You will receive these medications orally to avoid or treat asthma attacks.

Bronchial thermoplastic

Bronchial thermoplastic can be a surgical technique used for severe asthma that hasn't improved with other treatments. In this technique, radiofrequency energy is put on the airway. The heat that's generated destroys a number of the smooth muscle lining on the airway. This prevents the muscle from constricting and narrowing the opening.

Bronchial thermoplastic is certainly delivered in three sessions, each given three weeks apart. Though it is not a cure for asthma, research shows it can reduce symptoms.

The Continuing Future of Severe Asthma Treatments

Researchers remain looking for new drugs that'll be in a position to prevent and relieve asthma symptoms. One drug, which has generated a whole lot of excitement is ***Fevipiprant (QAW039).*** Though yet in development, this experimental drug reduced symptoms and improved lung function in people who have allergic asthma that inhaled *corticosteroids* couldn't control. If *Fevipiprant* is approved, it might be the first fresh oral asthma drug for being introduced in twenty years.

Different studies are investigating the factors that are likely involved in asthma development. Identifying the triggers that tripped asthma symptoms could One (1) day enable researchers to avoid those processes preventing asthma before it starts.

Chapter 7

Complications of Unmanaged Asthma

The problem is treatable if a sign isn't resulting in other health issues.

There are numerous effective treatments for asthma that will help you manage your symptoms and continue with daily activities. At some times, however, asthma might be challenging to regulate if it remains poorly controlled, which might happen if you're not pursuing your prescribed treatment solution. Or it might be because your asthma is severe enough that your symptoms can't be managed by standard therapies, which typically include a long-term controller and quick-relief medications.

In addition to presenting an elevated risk to get more bothersome symptoms and attacks, people who have uncontrolled asthma likewise have a higher threat of other significant health complications. Included in these are:

- **Reduced ability to participate in typical day to**

day activities, symptoms of asthma-like coughing, wheezing, and shortness of breathing might lead to you being sick and tired of work or college, affecting your productivity. Asthma symptoms could also interfere with rest or prevent you from working out or participating in other leisure or interpersonal activities, which might affect your current health and boost your risk for conditions like cardiovascular disease and diabetes. A cross-sectional evaluation released in March 2017 in NPJ Main Care Respiratory Medication found that individuals who have poorly managed asthma were much more likely to see work and overall activity impairments than individuals who have asthma in order.

- **Severe asthma attacks:** According to a report published in Sept 2018 in the journal Advances in Therapy, up to 10 percent of people who've asthma could have a severe type that's difficult to regulate, which can increase their risk for potentially life-threatening attacks. Whoever has experienced an unrelenting asthma assault understands how scary they could be. A critical asthma strike could cause severe breathlessness or wheeze with difficulty talking blue lip area or fingernails, or other symptoms that don't improve after taking your medication.

Pursuing your asthma treatment solution should assist in preventing attacks, though your symptoms may still flare up sometimes. However, if you're not keeping to your recommended treatment or if it isn't working well for your asthma, your experience of attack may be severe enough to result in a visit to the (ER) or require hospitalization. A study of individuals with asthma in the U.S. and U.K. released in Apr 2017 in the journal BMC Pulmonary Medication found that those people who have a brief history of severe asthma episodes that require medical assistance are roughly doubly likely to go to the ER or need medical center services for his or her asthma in the foreseeable future than those people who have never experienced severe episodes.

- **Airway remodeling:** When you have asthma, your airways become inflamed, which in turn causes these to swell and produce extra mucus. Unless this swelling has been effectively treated, it can eventually lead to a long term narrowing of the bronchial pipes in your lungs, Dr. Rosenstreich says. This so-called *"airway redesigning"* is irreversible and makes a difference to how you breathe. Some individuals may eventually need to use an assistive device, as an air machine, to inhale. It's believed that everyone that has asthma encounters airway modeling to some extent; however, severe *airway remodeling* is uncommon. "When irritation in the lungs isn't properly managed by therapy with corticosteroids or bronchodilators, scar tissue formation can develop, and the airways are no more able to start, even after using an inhaler." "It could begin soon after the starting point of asthma, which explains why I encourage visitors to adhere to their recommended therapy."

- **Unwanted effects of long-term use of certain medications:** As regards Asthma Australia, the medial side results associated with corticosteroid and bronchodilator treatment are rare and, generally, small. Though, the use of inhalers could cause a loud tone of voice or fungal attacks in the mouth area.

"Unwanted effects are less normal with inhaled medications because the active component remains in the airway or is rapidly metabolized once it enters the bloodstream."

However, with oral corticosteroids, you might experience side effects such as *disturbed sleep, hyperactivity, and increased appetite. Long-term use of dental corticosteroids may boost your risk of attacks, high blood sugars, and osteoporosis.*

Speak to your doctor if you're experiencing any side effects – and you shouldn't stop taking asthma medication without your doctor's authorization.

- **Stress and depression:** Much like many chronic diseases, having asthma may boost your risk for anxiety and depression. A report of adults who've asthma in Korea released in the May-June 2017 problem of Asthma and Allergy Proceedings discovered that those who got asthma were almost twice as more likely to develop depression as those without the problem.

"A disorder like asthma can have a substantial mental toll." If you're sense depressed or stressed, speak to your doctor to make sure you get the treatment you will need. "Asthma can be considered a problem, but it's manageable."

- **The higher threat of developing gastroesophageal reflux disease (GERD):** An article published in Dec 2013 in the journal *Scientifica* shows that approximately 80 percent of individuals who've asthma symptoms of GERD, or acid reflux disorder - and it's more prevalent in those people who have hard-to-control asthma than in those whose asthma is well-controlled. Research also indicates that GERD may get worse asthma symptoms and additionally reduce the performance of treatment.

"There's some proof that the bronchodilators used to take care of asthma may promote acidity creation in the belly and regurgitation in the esophagus." If you begin to see acid reflux, make sure to speak to your doctor.

- **Obstructive Sleep Apnoea (OSA)**

The same *Scientifica* review notes that risk for OSA, which can cause snoring and breathing difficulties while asleep, is almost doubly high among individuals who have asthma than it is within those without the problem.

- **Pneumonia and other respiratory infections**

Asthma itself doesn't boost your risk for pneumonia or other styles of lung attacks. However, a report published in Dec 2013 in the journal Upper body found that individuals who used the highest-strength inhaled corticosteroids to take care of asthma were more than doubly apt to be identified as having pneumonia or another lower respiratory system contamination than the healthy control topics, which can be because of the use of inhalers that aren't properly washed, or because the corticosteroids, while reducing swelling, inhibit some common disease fighting capability function.

"These infections are a problem by using any anti-inflammatory." Individuals who use inhalers can also experience fungal attacks in the mouth area. "That's why it's important to wash out the mouth area with water or mouthwash after making use of your inhaler."

How to Lessen the Threat of Complications

In general, dealing with your doctor can support you in finding the correct treatment to regulate your asthma symptoms and lessen your risk of complications. And, once you find a cure that works for you, it's essential to stay with it.

"A lot of people with asthma know the need for staying on recommended treatment." "Because if indeed they don't, they know they'll see a rise in their symptoms. However, your doctor will remind you that symptoms are just the beginning. These problems are, generally, uncommon, and avoidable, by just sticking to your treatment."

Though if you have trouble controlling your symptoms despite following your treatment solution, ask your doctor if you might have a far more severe form of asthma, such as *eosinophilic asthma*. You will find newer medications open to treat this kind of asthma, which is designated by high degrees of inflammation-causing white bloodstream cells called eosinophils in the lungs - and a significant change in treatment can help you control your symptoms and stop related health problems.

Chapter 8

Natural Remedies for Managing Asthma

When you have severe asthma, as well as your standard medications are not providing the relief you will need, you might be curious whether there are other things you should do to handle your symptoms.

Some natural treatments might be able to ease your symptoms, decrease the amount of medication you will need to use, and generally enhance the quality you will ever have. These remedies work best when taken alongside your usual prescribed asthma medications.

Listed below are 13 complementary therapies you can test and also asthma.

1. Dietary changes

Although there is no specific diet for those who have severe asthma, there are many actions you can take that might help with your symptoms.

Being overweight could worsen severe asthma. It is

essential to maintain a wholesome and balanced diet, which includes *plenty of vegetables & fruits*. These are sound resources of antioxidants like **beta-carotene** and **vitamins C** and **E**, plus they can help to lessen inflammation around your airways.

If you experience an upsurge in asthma symptoms after eating particular foods, stay away from eating them. It may be a food allergy that is causing your symptoms to worsen. Speak to your doctor to verify this.

2. Buteyko Breathing Technique

The Buteyko Breathing Technique (BBT) is something of breathing exercises. It would be able to lessen your asthma symptoms through slow, gentle breathing.

BBT targets breathing out of your respective nose rather than the mouth area. Breathing out of the mouth area can dry your airways and make sure they are more sensitive.

Some individuals may experience fewer respiratory infections from using this system. Other people who practice BBT think that it can help to improve your skin tightening and levels. Still, there is no conclusive evidence to aid this theory.

3. Papworth method

The Papworth method is a breathing and relaxation technique that is used in the 1960s to help people who have asthma greatly. It involves making use of your nose and diaphragm to build up breathing patterns. After that, you can apply these breathing patterns to various activities that could cause your asthma to flare-up.

An exercise course is normally recommended before adopting the exercises in your daily routine.

4. Garlic

Garlic has countless health advantages, including anti-inflammatory diseases, according to some 2013 analysis. Because asthma can be an inflammatory disease, garlic would be able to help relieve your symptoms.

Still, there is no conclusive evidence that garlic works well against preventing an asthma attack.

5. Ginger

Ginger is another herb that has anti-inflammatory properties and could assist with severe asthma. A 2013 study showed that oral ginger supplements were associated with a noticeable difference in asthma symptoms. Nonetheless, it didn't concur that ginger triggers a noticeable difference in overall lung function.

6. Honey

Honey is generally found in cold remedies to help soothe throat and reduce coughing significantly. You may mix honey using a hot beverage like herbal tea to help relieve symptoms.

Nonetheless, there are limited Trusted Source scientific evidence that Honey ought to be used as asthma treatment alternatively.

7. Omega-3 oils

Omega-3 oils that exist in *fish* and *flax seeds* have already been shown to hold many health advantages. They could also work to diminish airway inflammation and improve lung function in people who have severe asthma. High doses of oral steroids, though, can block the beneficial effects of omega-3 oils. It's wise to check with your doctor before boosting your intake of omega-3.

8. Caffeine

Caffeine can be a bronchodilator and may reduce respiratory muscle fatigue. A 2010 study from a Trusted Source showed that caffeine could be effective for those who have asthma. It would be able to enhance the function of airways for four hours after consumption.

9. Yoga

Yoga incorporates stretching and breathing exercises to help boost flexibility and boost your general health fitness significantly. For many individuals, practicing yoga can decrease stress, which may trigger your asthma.

The breathing techniques employed in yoga also may help to lessen the frequency of asthma attacks. However, there is not currently any conclusive evidence to prove this.

10. Hypnotherapy

In hypnotherapy, hypnosis can be used to make a person additionally relaxed and available to new methods of thinking, feeling, and behavior. Hypnotherapy can help facilitate muscle relaxation, which might help people who have asthma deal with symptoms like chest tightness.

11. Mindfulness

Mindfulness is a kind of meditation that targets the way the mind and your body are sense in today's moment. It could be used almost anywhere. All that you'll require is a quiet spot to sit back, close your eyes, and concentrate on the thoughts, feelings, and sensations within you.

Due to its stress-relieving benefits, mindfulness can help complement your prescription drugs and relieve stress-related asthma symptoms.

12. Acupuncture

Acupuncture is a kind of ancient Chinese medicine which involves placing small needles into specific points on your body. Long-term great things about acupuncture never have yet shown to work against asthma. However, many people who have asthma do discover that acupuncture helps to improve airflow and manage symptoms like chest pain.

13. Pelotherapy

Speleotherapy involves hanging out inside a salt room to introduce tiny particles of salt into the respiratory system. There happens to be no scientific evidence to prove that speleotherapy is an efficient type of treatment against asthma. Still, one study from a Trusted Source did show it had a beneficial influence on short-term lung function.

Chapter 9

Natural Solution to Asthma

Asthma can be a chronic lung condition that triggers difficulty breathing. The airways from the lungs, called bronchial tubes, become inflamed. The encompassing muscles tighten, and mucus is produced, which further narrows the airways. Untreated asthma attacks can result in hospitalization and may even come to be fatal. It isn't a problem that needs to be self-treated.

Symptoms and Signs

Asthma symptoms can range between mild, such as wheezing, to chronic coughing and wheezing during severe asthma attacks. They are several indicators and symptoms:

- *Wheezing and shortness of breath,*

- *Difficulty sleeping because of shortness of breath, wheezing and coughing,*

- *Chest pain or tightness,*

- *Shortness of breath during exercise.*

NB: *Self-treating and avoiding or delaying standard care may have serious consequences.*

Natural Remedies

Below is a list of natural remedies to contain the severity of asthma attack from home;

1) Buteyko Breathing Technique

The **Buteyko** (pronounced as *bew-tay-ko*) **Breathing Technique** originated by Russian-born researcher *Konstantin Pavlovich Buteyko*. It includes shallow breathing exercises made to help people who have asthma breathe easily.

The Buteyko Breathing Technique is dependant on the premise that raising blood degrees of skin tightening and through shallow breathing might help people who have asthma. Skin tightening and is thought to dilate the smooth muscles on the airways.

A report involving 60 people who have asthma compared the consequences on the *Buteyko Breathing Technique*, a tool that mimics **pranayama** (*a yoga breathing technique*), and a *placebo*. Researchers found people while using the *Buteyko Breathing Technique* had a decrease in asthma symptoms. Symptoms didn't change in the pranayama as well as the placebo groups.

The usage of inhalers was low in the Buteyko group by two puffs a trip to half a year, but there is no change in the different two groups.

Other promising clinical trials were evaluated; however, they have already been small in proportions and will experience other issues with the analysis design. Critics with the technique say that the method is expensive, that it creates no difference in the quantity of skin tightening and inside the blood, that higher degrees of skin tightening and is not a highly effective strategy, which any effect of the technique could be because of general relaxation.

2) Omega-3 Essential Oil

Among the primary inflammation-causing fats inside our diets is thought to be *arachidonic acid*. Arachidonic acid is situated in particular foods, such as *egg yolks, shellfish, and meat*. Consuming less of the meals is considered to decrease inflammation and asthma symptoms.

"A German study examined data from 524 children and discovered that asthma was more frequent in children with high degrees of arachidonic acid."

Arachidonic acid may also be produced in our anatomies. Another technique to reduce degrees of arachidonic acid is definitely to improve the intake of essential oil such as *EPA (eicosapentaenoic acid) from fish oil* and *GLA (gamma-linolenic acid)* from borage or *evening primrose oil*.

Omega-3 oil capsules can be purchased in drug stores, health food stores, and online. Search for the substances in **EPA** and **DHA** in the label. To lessen a fishy aftertaste of using fish oil capsules, they must be taken a right before meals.

Omega-3 oil capsules may interact with blood-thinning drugs such as warfarin *(Coumadin) and aspirin.* Side effects can include *indigestion and bleeding.*

3) Vegetables & fruits

A report examining food diaries of 68,535 women discovered that women who had a larger intake of *tomatoes, carrots, and leafy vegetables* had less prevalence of asthma.

High consumption of apples may drive back asthma. Daily intake of fruits & vegetables in childhood lowered the chance of asthma.

A University of Cambridge study discovered that asthma symptoms in adults are connected with *minimal dietary intake of fruit, vitamin C, and manganese.*

4) Butterbur

Butterbur can be a perennial shrub that expands in

Europe, Asia, and The United States. The active constituents are *petasin and isopetasin*, which are thought to reduce smooth muscle spasm and also have an anti-inflammatory effect.

Researchers at the University of Dundee, Scotland, evaluated the consequences of butterbur in people who have allergic asthma who had also been using inhalers. They discovered that butterbur put into the anti-inflammatory aftereffect of the inhalers.

Another analysis examined the usage of the *butterbur root extract* in 80 people who have asthma for four months. The quantity, duration, and severity of asthma attacks decreased, and symptoms improved after using butterbur. A lot more than 40 percent of individuals using asthma medication at the beginning of the report reduced their intake of drugs by the end of the analysis.

Side effects of butterbur can include indigestion, headache, fatigue, nausea, vomiting, diarrhea, or constipation. Pregnant or nursing women, children, or people who have kidney or liver disease shouldn't take butterbur.

Butterbur is in the ragweed plant family, so *people who are allergic to ragweed, marigold, daisy, or chrysanthemum shouldn't take butterbur.*

The raw herb, as well as teas, extracts, and capsules created from the natural herb shouldn't be used because they contain substances called *pyrrolizidine alkaloids* that may be toxic towards the liver and kidneys and also have been associated with cancer.

You would need to take away the pyrrolizidine alkaloids from butterbur products. For instance, in Germany, there's a safety limit to the number of pyrrolizidine alkaloids allowed in butterbur products. The daily recommended dose cannot exceed *one microgram each day.*

5) Bromelain

Bromelain is an extract from pineapples. Among the theories about how exactly it works is that it's thought to have anti-inflammatory features. In one analysis, researchers at the University of Connecticut discovered that bromelain reduced airway inflammation in animals with allergic airway disease. Bromelain shouldn't be used by people who have allergies to pineapples.

Side effects can include digestive upset and allergies.

6) Boswellia

The herb *Boswellia*, known in *Indian Ayurvedic medicine* as **Salai guggul**, continues to be within preliminary studies to inhibit the forming of compounds called leukotrienes. Leukotrienes released in the lungs cause narrowing of airways.

A double-blind, placebo-controlled study of forty patients, 40 people who have asthma, were treated having a Boswellia extract three (3) times every day for six weeks. By the end of the period, 70 percent of individuals had improved. Symptoms of difficulty breathing, the number of attacks, and laboratory measures had improved.

Boswellia comes in pill type. It should declare on the

label that it's standardized to contain 60 percent *Boswellia acids*. It would not be used for a lot more than 8 to 12 weeks unless otherwise recommended by a professional health practitioner.

It isn't crystal clear what dose is safe or effective or how Boswellia may interact with additional asthma treatments. *Side effects may include digestive upset, nausea, acid reflux disorder, or diarrhea.*

7) Weight Loss

Numerous studies have discovered that obesity can be a risk factor for asthma.

8) Biofeedback

Biofeedback may also be recommended by practitioners as an all-natural therapy for asthma.

Caveats

Supplements have never been tested for safety, and

because health supplements are mostly unregulated, this content of some products varies from what's specified on the merchandise label.

Also, take into account that the safety of supplements in women that are pregnant, nursing mothers, children, and the ones with medical ailments or who are taking medications is not established.

Chapter 10
Medications for Asthma

Medications play an integral role in how you control your ailment. A couple of the main types of treatment each aimed toward a particular goal are;

- ✓ **Controller medications:** They are the most crucial because they prevent asthma episodes. By using these drugs, your airways are less swollen and less inclined to react to causes.

- ✓ **Quick-relief medications:** also known as rescue medications, relax the muscles around your airway. When you have to use a rescue medication more than twice weekly, your asthma isn't well-controlled. But individuals who have Exercise-induced Asthma might use a quick-acting med called a beta-alpha before a good work out.

The proper medication should enable you to live an active and healthy life. In case your asthma symptoms aren't managed, ask your doctor to support you in finding a different treatment that increases results.

✓ **Long-Term Control Medications**

A few of these drugs should be studied daily to get your asthma in order and keep it that way. Others are used as a needed basis to lessen the severity of the asthma attack.

The very best ones stop airway inflammation. Your doctor may suggest you combine an inhaled corticosteroid, an anti-inflammatory medication with other drugs such as:

- *Long-acting beta-agonists:*

  A beta-alpha is a kind of medicine called a ***bronchodilator,*** which helps your airways.

- *Long-acting anticholinergics:*

  Anticholinergics relax and enlarge (dilate) the airways in the lungs, making respiration easier (***bronchodilators***).

- ***Tiotropium bromide (Spiriva Respimat):*** can be

an *anticholinergic* designed for anyone aged range six and older. This medication should be utilized in addition to your regular maintenance medication.

- ***Leukotriene modifiers:*** it stops chemicals that cause swelling. *Mast cell stabilizers* curb the discharge of chemicals that causes inflammation.

- ***Theophylline:*** is a bronchodilator used as an add-on medication for symptoms that aren't answering to other medicines.

- ***An immunomodulator:*** can be a shot given if you have moderate to severe asthma-related allergies or other irritation caused by the disease fighting capability that doesn't react to certain drugs.

- ***Reslizumab (Cinqair):*** can be an immunomodulator-maintenance medication. It is utilized with your regular asthma medications. This medication is given every four weeks as an intravenous shot for about one hour. This medication functions by reducing the amount of a particular kind of white bloodstream cells, called *eosinophil(s)*, which are likely involved in leading to asthma symptoms. It could reduce severe asthma episodes.

- ***Mepolizumab (Nucala:)*** focuses on the degrees of bloodstream eosinophil(s). It is given as a shot every four weeks and can be used as a maintenance therapy medication.

- ***Omalizumab (Xolair):*** can be an antibody that blocks *immunoglobulin E (IgE)* and is used as an asthma management medication, which prevents an allergen from triggering an asthma strike. This medication is given as a shot. To get this medicine for one with a raised IgE level and also has known allergy symptoms. The allergies have to be verified by either bloodstream or epidermis test.

www.ingramcontent.com/pod-product-compliance
Lightning Source LLC
Chambersburg PA
CBHW071114030426
42336CB00013BA/2073